MW00947026

FLOURISH!

The Method Used by Aging Services Organizations
for the Ultimate Marketing Results

By Wendy O'Donovan Phillips

Copyright © 2018 O'Donovan Phillips
All rights reserved.

To all of the professionals in aging services,
for all that you give.

And to Dad, my anchor.

TABLE OF CONTENTS

FROM MYSTERY TO METHOD

Alan Wyngarden started with an extraordinary vision for his aging services organization. He set out to create an assisted living and memory care community that welcomes residents to feel at home.

Today, Alan's vision is a reality. His homes are designed as if the residents bought them for their very own family. Team members are genuine, accepting and caring. They get face-to-face and heart-to-heart with residents, creating an intimate environment where seniors thrive. The care team makes a conscious effort to validate each resident, whether that means sitting and listening to their stories, or encouraging them to set the table and participate in the various tasks of the home.

There's only one problem.

Alan became over-invested in referral agencies, spending hundreds of thousands of dollars for new leads that rarely converted into residents. He and his marketing team had plenty of marketing tactics, but no real strategy.

Quietly, Alan's potential residents were leaking away to the competition. As hard as everyone worked, they became disheartened.

Alan is not alone. Senior living communities everywhere are increasingly bogged down by the frustrations of marketing. The competition is brutal, and it seems nearly impossible these days to differentiate in a sea of sameness. What's more, it's an uphill battle to attract and retain passionate team members who make an organization thrive.

Unfortunately, conventional thinking prevails. Online marketing is all the rage these days, so why not try a little of that? Clients and families occasionally refer, but how do we attract high-quality referrals on a regular basis? Does the website need to be updated, or are marketing dollars best invested elsewhere? Oh well, the marketing is working okay. Hopefully inquiries will come.

Hope is not a method. Here is the precise method to marketing:

1. Survey the clients, families and team
2. Define a Message and Design Equation
3. Build a Balanced Marketing Formula
4. Deploy the plan for steadfast results

Welcome to the *FLOURISH!* method. It's how I worked with Alan to unite his vision with his revenue goals. We put into writing a baseline of where he was and where he wanted to be in 12 months. I asked him about his residents and those families who believed in his vision.

I surveyed his residents, families and team members with a questionnaire to find out what they appreciated about his community. In the process, they revealed how they went about finding his community, and which competitors they considered. Then I looked closely at those competitors to see what they were delivering. I shared what I learned with Alan.

His residents and families had shared stories of transformation. Alan and his team were *changing lives.* And these stories were marketing gold.

From the written survey responses, we defined exactly the *message* that resonated best with residents and families, to target new residents. We articulated that message in writing. We then put to paper what *design* best matched that message. Together, these two tools became the Message and Design Equation. These tools helped us stay consistent in how his community's marketing spoke, looked and felt.

Next we built a Balanced Marketing Formula, or marketing plan. Based upon the survey results, Alan and I collaborated on how to tell the unique story about his community and differentiate his from the others. We set out to attract his target audience: seniors with memory care needs and their families. We agreed to deploy just three tactics in his Balanced Marketing Formula:

1. Redevelop the *website* with improved messaging, design and layout
2. Launch a robust *sales* campaign to attract residents
3. Ratchet up his word-of-mouth family *referrals*

That's it. Just three tactics re-energized his community with a *strategic* formula for success. And we had the data to back it.

Over the months that followed we put the Balanced Marketing Formula to work.

And it worked!

The *FLOURISH!* method helped Alan fulfill his vision and keep occupancies high at his community.

The *FLOURISH!* method has helped countless more aging services organizations validate their marketing efforts. They enjoy higher returns on marketing investments, more stability and steady growth. The method is based on research and results with hundreds of aging services organizations over the years. Organizations like Alan's. Organizations like yours.

Are you ready to put the *FLOURISH!* method to work for your organization?

HOW TO USE THIS BOOK

This book is ideal for anyone handling marketing for any aging services organization, including but not limited to: life plan communities, independent living communities, assisted living communities, memory support communities, skilled nursing and long-term care communities, home health and home care services, adult day services and hospice organizations.

There are three ways to get the most out of this book, independent of each other or blended:

1. **Do-It-Yourself Guide.** If you want total control and prefer to create the marketing, execute the *FLOURISH!* method yourself. Follow the step-by-step instructions for everything needed to be successful, with occasional help from outsiders.

2. **Marketing Handbook.** Perhaps you have a marketing team. In that case, train the frontline staff on the exercises at the end of the book to lay the foundation for the *FLOURISH!* method. Once that's in place, leave the creation and delivery of the marketing to your team, using the method as a guide.

3. **Litmus Test.** Maybe you prefer to outsource the marketing to an agency and focus your team exclusively on nurturing warm leads. In that case, use the *FLOURISH!* method to test whether the agency's solutions really work.

The detailed approach of these lessons will help hold them accountable.

4. **Hit the Reset Button.** Perhaps the marketing team has gotten off-center in following brand standards, efficiently getting promotional initiatives to market or reaching sales goals. The *FLOURISH!* method is a great refresher for getting everyone back on track and reaching goals.

Before I started my own marketing agency, I was employed by another firm where I got to work on big accounts like Microsoft and Wells Fargo. I learned the strategies Fortune 500 companies nationwide deploy to ensure high returns and solid results from their marketing. I distilled those strategies down to their most essential parts to deliver them to smaller entities, namely in the healthcare sector.

This book outlines those strategies.

What you will read here is not rocket science. You will see these basic strategies in play daily, even in your own life. Your phone, computer, social media pages, even your barista – are all constantly gathering data to understand what you like most about their product or service. From that data, companies are diminishing the aspects you don't prefer, and delivering more of the traits you do prefer. This is how they make you a loyal and referring customer.

This concept is the overarching theme of the *FLOURISH!* method. You may have never thought to put a science behind your organization's marketing. Or yours just might be a Fortune 500 company, but one that needs to refine and refocus marketing efforts.

Either way, now you can.

PART ONE

THE FOUNDATION OF THE *FLOURISH!* METHOD

The method starts with surveying the clients, families and team. It proceeds by defining a Message and Design Equation, then building a Balanced Marketing Formula as a 12-month marketing plan. Once this foundation is set, you will be well equipped to launch your marketing, tactic by tactic. Let's begin.

SURVEY THE CLIENTS, FAMILIES AND TEAM

The first step is to ask the right questions to understand how clients, families and the team think about the organization and how they consume marketing. An emailed survey looks simple yet provides immense insight. This section will detail how to effectively survey.

Why bother to survey? When you survey the clients, families and team, you get timely, relevant and actionable feedback. You learn precisely what they love most about the organization, and it's typically not the things that come to mind first. It's not standard of care. It's not philosophy. It's not even specialty. The thing they love best is the fact that *your organization makes life better.*

When surveyed correctly, respondents light up and share animated stories. Only the clients, families and team have the passion behind the story, and that passion surfaces when they start talking. A bunch of marketers couldn't make this stuff up alone.

Here's Alan's mission statement: "We provide an entire continuum of care by partnering with our residents and families to develop personalized nutrition plans, professionally developed geriatric exercise, mind stimulation and meaningful activities."

By contrast, here is how one of his happiest resident's family members talks about what his community does best: "You take care of my father in a caring, compassionate manner. The care team has gotten to know him and is perceptive to his every need. They keep him safe and make him feel like family. You are welcoming and helpful. You are love!"

Those who work in administrative roles for the organization, like the marketing team, tend to talk about features rather than benefits. Happy clients and families, on the other hand, delve into what's in it for them. They talk about how you changed their lives. This simply delights their friends and family, who then send more potential clients through warm referrals.

The survey extracts these stories so you can bottle them and put them to market. Nothing sells the organization like these stories.

This strategy goes beyond sprinkling a few testimonials here and there. These stories become the foundation of every marketing message.

The surveys also reveal what media is best to find the right audience. This is important to know so you invest time and money only in the marketing tactics that will help the organization succeed *now*. For example, if you discover your clients, families and the people they know aren't following Facebook, then don't invest there. But if every family reads the neighborhood newspaper cover-to-cover, run a print ad there. If 70% of the target audience pays attention to direct mail, then do that.

How to Survey
First, compile a list of favorite clients, families and team members: no fewer than 30 people and no more than 100. Include on the list family members who visit often, who articulate their needs and who cherish your approach. Include short-

term guests who participate in physical and occupational therapy as well as those family members who see the results of your efforts. They already respect your personalized engagement, clinical expertise, prompt attention to their needs and follow-up. These are people who you want to replicate because they produce a happy environment.

Next, craft the questions carefully for the survey. Here are a few to start:

- What are we doing best?
- What other aging services organizations did you consider?
- How are we different from those organizations?
- Would you refer friends and family to our organization?
- If so, what would encourage you to do so more often?
- Would you search online for an organization like this one?
- If so, what search terms would you use?
- What social media sites do you frequent?
    - o Facebook
    - o Instagram
    - o Twitter
    - o Other _____
- What types of marketing grab your attention?
    - o Website
    - o Online search
    - o Online ads
    - o Social media
    - o Online reviews
    - o Direct mail
    - o TV/radio
    - o Billboards
    - o Print ads

Customize the questions and corresponding choices to uncover information that will put marketing into action.

Some people forgo this exercise and jump directly to launching marketing tactics. Think again.

Lisa Stemmer of the medical device agency Ubiquity uses a similar survey and interview process to formulate targeted marketing plans. "Doing the homework first will save time and money," she explains. "If you have done your research to find your strategy, you will hit the target rather than shoot in the dark."

Marketing without strategy is a leaky cauldron. Stemmer says, "You lose two weeks here, two months there from your marketing efforts. Consider how many new leads, how much revenue, could have entered in that time with more focus. This brings to light the sheer cost of a lack of focus."

For example, says Stemmer, "We got a call from a client who had what I call a bright-shiny-object moment. She had suddenly decided a brochure was The Thing she needed to jumpstart her revenues. Trouble was, the brochure had absolutely no relationship to the vision and goals. I told the client, 'You are doing this for the sheer pleasure of yourself.'"

Marketing just for the sake of marketing seldom works. It's better to market in the name of attracting new inquiries. The most important part: "Once you have created the strategy, you have to embrace it," says Stemmer. "Referring back to it and marketing with consistency will bring the value, not just having it."

If you truly want to grow with a steady flow of the *right* leads, strategy is the only way to start. "It's like scrubbing in before surgery," says Stemmer. "It's the fundamental start to a complicated procedure."

Surveying early and often allows you to go to market with a message representing the essence of the organization. Eventually it becomes a self-fulfilling prophecy. It allows you to make the same promise across all tactics within the overall marketing strategy. It's the one promise that can be fulfilled every day, the one promise the organization becomes known for – the promise that clients and families know you will deliver.

Since the promise is derived from answers to questions like, "What are we doing best?" the promise can be articulated in the authentic words of clients and families. This way it resonates with potential clients and families who want to know you better. From the moment they enter the organization, the entire experience delivers on the promise made to them. Not only will they become loyal, but they will also tell others about the organization.

And that cycle means higher occupancies, higher revenues, higher profits and happier clients and families – all benefits of the *FLOURISH!* method.

CONSTRUCT THE MARKETING MESSAGE AND DESIGN EQUATION

Once you have asked the right questions of the right people, you will have the data needed to construct a Message and Design Equation exclusive to your aging services organization.

The verbatim survey responses lead to the Message and Design Equation. The equation articulates in writing and images what clients and families love most about the organization.

The equation is: Messaging + Design = Brand.

The brand is the biggest benefit you are best known for. Volvo is best known as "safe." Coca-Cola is best known as "refreshing." Geico is best known for "savings."

What is your organization best known for?

Branding is top-of-mind awareness. When you think of tissues, does Kleenex come to mind? When you think of copying, does Xerox pop up? There is a reason for that. Those companies have invested millions in helping us recall their name for a particular need at the moment we need it.

You don't need a million-dollar budget to do the same. Here's how to formulate the Message and Design Equation. The key is to depend on the survey results, not thoughts and feelings. Consider bringing in an objective third party to assist.

Look back through the survey responses for commonalities and trends. Based on those patterns, now complete the worksheet that appears at the end of the book – **Exercise 1: Your Message and Design Equation.**

- List three ways survey respondents say this organization is different and better than competitors.
- What is the No. 1 trait respondents like best about the organization?

As you write down the answer to the first question, the answer to the second one will emerge. The answer to the second question is the Message.

Now ask yourself, "What does this Message look like when translated into Design?"

Here are a few examples.

Example 1

What are three ways survey respondents say this organization is different and better than competitors?
- o Calm and comfort
- o Involved and engaged
- o Personalized care

What is the No. 1 trait respondents like best about the organization?
- o This community welcomes residents to feel at home again.

Message: "Welcome Home Again"
Design: Warm, comforting images of home

Example 2

What are three ways survey respondents say this organization is different and better than competitors?

- o Just like home
- o Genuinely interested and caring
- o As much independence as possible

What is the No. 1 trait respondents like best about the organization?

- o This community is where happiness comes to life

Message: "Happiness Comes to Life"

Design: Images of residents smiling and laughing

Example 3

What are three ways survey respondents say this organization is different and better than competitors?

- o True confidence
- o Around the clock care
- o Exceptional value

What is the No. 1 trait respondents like best about the organization?

- o This home-care service offers maximum peace of mind – right in your own neighborhood

Message: "Maximum Peace of Mind"

Design: Images of older adults and care partners in trusting interactions (a hand on a hand, an arm around the shoulder, eye-to-eye, etc.)

Once you have articulated the Message and Design Equation in the exercise at the end of the book, it remains fixed in place unless the organization changes. If, for example, another organization is acquired or the existing entity expands into new locations, then run the survey again and redevelop a new Message and Design Equation based upon new results.

The Message and Design Equation is an internal tool. It's not something the public will see, but a guide for how the marketing materials should read and look. The Message and Design Equation becomes the starting point for *everything* created to market the organization. This way, everything says the same thing and reflects a steady image. Repetition is what makes the unique story memorable.

Now that the Message and Design Equation is locked in, it's time to build the Balanced Marketing Formula for optimum results.

BUILD A BALANCED MARKETING FORMULA

Congratulations! You now have a Marketing and Design Equation, which is more than most aging services organizations ever do in terms of a marketing method. Now, let's take your strategy a step further.

The Balanced Marketing Formula is simply the marketing plan that outlines a handful of appropriate tactics to take your Message and Design Equation to market. The Balanced Marketing Formula earns higher returns than typical marketing plans because it caters to the target audience's media consumption behaviors. It disperses the marketing budget across all four strategies to drive new inquiries:

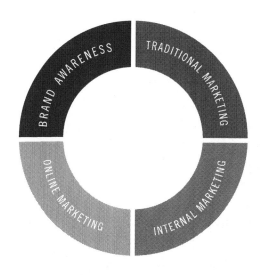

In senior living marketing, there are nearly 50 possible market tactics:

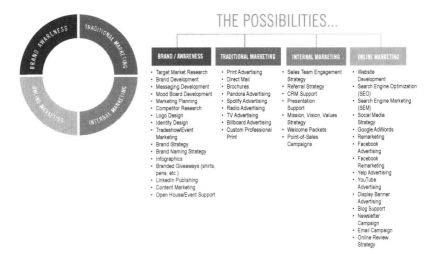

From the survey results, you now know what tactics resonate with your clients and families. Just look back over the answers to the question, "What types of marketing grab your attention?" Only a handful of highly targeted marketing tactics will be the focus over the next 12 months. Let the surveys indicate which ones.

Let's build upon the previous examples.

Example 1
Message and Design Equation:
"Welcome Home Again" +
Warm, comforting images of home
Balanced Marketing Formula:

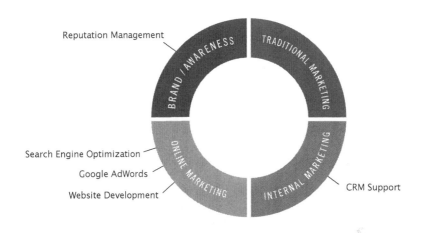

How do we know this is the right Balanced Marketing Formula for this organization? 38% of survey respondents initially became involved with the organization through an on-line search, and 100% believe their peers would search online for an organization like this one. Therefore, the community knew it had to improve its online presence with a new web-site. 75% of respondents said they would seek a referral from a friend, family member or doctor when looking for an aging services organization. Hence, a robust sales support strategy was launched, including investment in customer management software (CRM) and presentation skills training. Finally, 50% of survey respondents used or would use the internet when seeking out a community like this one. So search engine opti-mization (SEO) and Google AdWords were also added.

Example 2
Message and Design Equation:
"Happiness Comes to Life"+
Images of residents smiling and laughing
Balanced Marketing Formula:

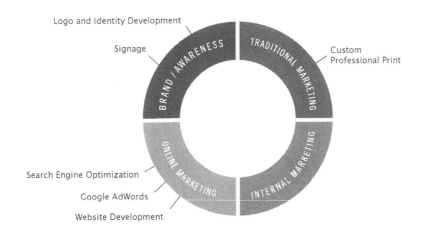

While this community's logo had certainly been updated since its founding in 1874, the surveys indicated it was time to refresh the logo, signage and print materials, as well as redesign the website. The surveys showed respondents would pay attention to online marketing, so search engine optimization (SEO) and Google AdWords commenced.

Example 3
Message and Design Equation:
"Maximum Peace of Mind" +
Images of older adults and care partners in trusting interactions
Balanced Marketing Formula:

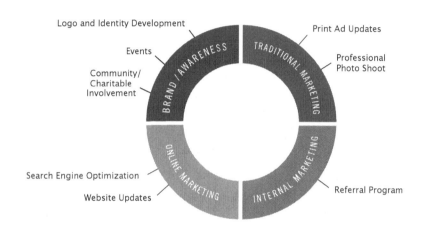

This home-care franchise had access to stock photos through the corporate office, but it needed more authentic photography for local marketing, images that would accurately represent the Message and Design Equation. With the survey results in hand, a few strategic updates to the local webpage were due, namely to align the text and imagery with the Message and Design Equation. Search engine optimization (SEO) would serve as a way to attract visitors to the website. A robust referral strategy would inspire clients and families to bring appropriate leads. Updated ad text would carry the message to the existing print medium, which survey respondents remembered well. Notably, the formula remains balanced across all four strategies of marketing.

Each Balanced Marketing Formula will look different because of factors like specialty, location, culture and vision. Marketing has to shift and grow with the organization.

The big thing that keeps marketing effective is the right Balanced Marketing Formula for your unique organization. It may look different next year than it did this year, depending upon shifting goals, trends and budget.

The Balanced Marketing Formula is composed of strategies and tactics that inevitably will overlap. The logo is part of brand awareness, and it will also appear in traditional media and online promotion. A referral program can evolve online just as well as offline. The welcome packet might be downloaded from the website or handed out in person.

Overlap is good. That way, you get the most mileage from effective marketing tactics. Rather than reinventing the wheel each time a marketing initiative is created, always ask, "How can this be used in multiple ways for a higher return on investment?"

Now, let's build your Balanced Marketing Formula.

Tactics
Begin by revisiting the survey responses to all the questions related to marketing tactics, such as these:

- Would you refer friends and family to our organization?
- If so, what would encourage you to do so more often?
- Would you search online for an organization like this one?
- If so, what search terms would you use?
- What social media sites do you frequent?
    - o Facebook
    - o Instagram
    - o Twitter
    - o Other _____
- What types of marketing grab your attention?
    - o Website
    - o Online search
    - o Online ads
    - o Social media
    - o Online reviews
    - o Direct mail
    - o TV/radio
    - o Billboards
    - o Print ads

Complete the exercise that appears at the end of the book – **Exercise 2: Your Balanced Marketing Formula** – with the names of tactics mentioned most often by your survey respondents.

***

Party Responsible
Now, write next to each tactic on your Balanced Marketing Formula the party responsible, or who will be in charge of executing or managing that tactic.

This is a simple yet critical step. To get any marketing tactic off the ground, it must be assigned to a capable and willing person or small group.

***

Marketing Budget
The next thing to complete on your Balanced Marketing Formula is the marketing budget.

Decide how much to budget for marketing for the year. This is typically 5% to 7% of annual revenue, but it can widely vary. Document your annual marketing budget in the designated area on the Balanced Marketing Formula.

Next, collect estimates from vendors, search out fees online and forecast costs with the marketing team, tactic by tactic. Write down the marketing budget for each tactic on the Balanced Marketing Formula.

Make no mistake, marketing is fluid. Because it's an ongoing investment, it should constitute a line item on the profit and loss report, just like payroll. And it's an investment, not just an expense. And any good investment yields healthy returns.

***

Expected ROI
The next step to completing the Balanced Marketing Formula is to forecast the expected ROI, or return on investment.

Consider each tactic's marketing budget on the Balanced Marketing Formula.

Then, estimate how many new inquires the Balanced Marketing Formula should attract. Ask each party responsible to provide projected new leads from each tactic. Document the projection on the line labeled "Expected ROI." Complete the exercise by multiplying the average value of a client by the projection of acquired clients, then subtracting the amount budgeted for this tactic. Document this dollar figure next to Expected ROI by tactic as well. Be sure to fill in the total annual Expected ROI, too, including total number of new clients and total dollar figure.

Now you are ready to execute the marketing tactics outlined on the Balanced Marketing Formula. Run all the tactics consistently for six months, and measure results before tweaking anything. As in any experiment, a baseline is needed before the discovery is observed. After the trial period, analyze the reports to see what to continue and what to fix or nix.

***

Actual ROI
The Balanced Marketing Formula is built to be successful, so be sure to measure that success.

Some general ways to measure success may include the organization's financial reporting or monthly census reports. In addition to being helpful in gauging the success of the total Balanced Marketing Formula, these reports can demonstrate the success of brand awareness and internal marketing strategies that are more difficult to measure alone.

For progress reports on online promotions, rely on Google Analytics reporting or other website analytics and social media analytics. Numerous YouTube videos detail how to get the most out of these reports.

For reporting on traditional media, rely on the vendors. Any reputable direct mail house will be able to provide relevant analytics on a campaign's performance. The same goes for newspaper and magazine representatives as well as television, radio and billboard account executives. Make them prove their success or cut them loose.

To get more granular in measuring actual ROI, consider including custom phone numbers to track calls from certain tactics. This will pinpoint what's working best and what needs fine-tuning.

Advise the team to always ask and document how new leads found the organization. If they are vague, ask probing questions to narrow the focus. "You say you saw it on the internet. On Google or Facebook?"

Determine the exact number of clients that came from each tactic. Document this in the actual ROI sections of the Balanced Marketing Formula, including actual ROI for each tactic as well as total actual ROI.

This will build a record of measurement to return to in six months. If the tactic worked, keep it. If not, alter it and test again. If it's still not working in another six months, replace it. But give it time, and be patient. While it may not catch on in month 6, it may take off in month 8.

***

Now you have surveyed clients, families and team memberss. You have constructed a Message and Design Equation and built a Balanced Marketing Formula. This is the foundation for the *FLOURISH!* method. These tools will allow you to experiment and get creative with marketing while still adhering to guidelines for success. This is the modern way to launch the most effective marketing tactics.

You are ready to deploy the Balanced Marketing Formula, tactic by tactic. Get ready for enduring results.

TOP 10 MISTAKES IN SETTING
THE FOUNDATION

1. **Experimenting without a hypothesis.** Instead, set a goal first. Expect the *FLOURISH!* method to produce measurable results such as an uptick in leads per month or in annual revenue. With a goal in mind, you can clearly measure success.

2. **Doing what's popular.** Rather than throwing money at online marketing because it's trendy, invest only in the marketing tactics that make most sense for your organization.

3. **Too many chefs in the kitchen.** Stick to two or three key decision-makers who will be with you throughout the whole process. Avoid crowdsourcing, which is gathering anecdotal opinions, as that can be more harmful than helpful in a strategic environment.

4. **Going it alone.** A lack of collaboration can be equally detrimental. Let the happiest clients and families tell the organization's story rather than trying to write it in a vacuum. This process will prevent you from getting too technical in your marketing communications. Plus, a small team of two or three colleagues will help you think creatively and stay on track.

5. **Re-experimenting too soon.** Once you discover the Balanced Marketing Formula, test those tactics for a good six months before changing or adding tactics. It takes that long to determine if the experiment is working. Patience, patience, patience!

6. **Letting your own opinion rule.** What clients and families think about the organization trumps what you think. Rely on their input to objectively build the Message and Design Equation.

7. **Feature focusing.** Turn your attention to benefits instead. Highlight what your clients and families love most about your organization, not meals and activities.

8. **Spending, not investing.** Be careful not to overspend on marketing. If after six months a tactic is not producing a return on investment, alter it. But keep in mind that returns are not always in the form of dollars. Added exposure and awareness in front of the people who matter most can be a very healthy investment. Again, adhere to the budget.

9. **Lack of documentation.** The foundation will erode – and fast – unless it's articulated in writing. Finish the exercises provided at the end of the book to be sure you have all the documentation you need for marketing success.

10. **Perfectionism.** Now that you have a method behind the marketing, there may be the tendency to overthink things. Set deadlines. Consider the idea that 80% done is done. Have a team member keep you accountable for finishing projects within a certain timeframe. And by the way, have fun!

PART TWO

BRAND AWARENESS

Now that you have completed the survey process, constructed a Message and Design Equation and built a Balanced Marketing Formula, it's time to deploy the marketing, tactic by tactic.

Part Two demonstrates how to deploy brand awareness tactics like logo, tagline and signage – if they appear in your Balanced Marketing Formula.

Brand awareness is all about staying "top of mind." When it comes to brand awareness efforts, it can be difficult to test each of these tactics, analyze data, draw conclusions and track results.

That's why it is critical that brand awareness tactics become part of the Balanced Marketing Formula, which will include more measurable tactics.

THE SCIENCE BEHIND THE LOGO

Maybe the survey responses revealed it's time to redesign the logo. If logo development is a tactic in your Balanced Marketing Formula, here are simple instructions on what to do.

Let's start with the anatomy of several types of logos:

1. **Custom Font Only** – FedEx is a well-known example. This font (or typeface) is memorable for its bold, blocky letters and it includes a hidden arrow to convey motion. The custom font is not the standard Arial or Times New Roman, but a unique typeface that stands for dependable shipping. There is nothing else to the logo other than the letters of the brand name. In the wellness world, Zantac, CVS Pharmacy and Johnson & Johnson are Custom Font Only logos. They work best for organizations with highly memorable names.

2. **Mark Plus Font** – Starbucks is the most ubiquitous example. We all know the white siren, or twin-tailed mermaid, that hearkens back to the coffeemaker's origins in seafaring Seattle. She appears inside of a green circle – that's the "mark." Around the mark originally appeared the words "Starbucks Coffee" – that's the font. (The company has dropped the words since the mark is now recognizable on its own, like the Target bullseye.) In healthcare, Blue Cross Blue Shield, Mayo Clinic and American Red Cross have Mark Plus Font logos. It's a great way for an organization to showcase brand through word and image.

3. **Initial Plus Font** – Everyone knows the McDonald's golden arches and the ubiquitous "M." The mark is the first initial of the brand name. Initial Plus Font logos in health and wellness include the universal blue "H" that provides roadside directions to hospitals, MALA for the Michigan Assisted Living Association and AARP for the American Association of Retired Persons. The Initial Plus Font logo is best for an organization that has a lot of brand equity built into its name; in other words, the name has been in use for many years and is easily recognized by the entire organization. Think NY for New York Yankees.

When it comes to choosing a font, there are numerous options. Notice that this book is written in a Serif Font, in which each letter has small lines or tiny feet on its end. Serif Fonts with feet are typically used in long-form writing because they are regarded as more legible for longer reading. Newspapers and magazines use Serif Fonts in their body copy. In a logo, a Serif Font can convey longevity and stability. It can also make a longer brand name easier to read. Favorite Serif Fonts for logos include:

Garamond

Baskerville

Georgia

By contrast, the fonts below use a Sans Serif Font. "Sans" is French for "without." The Sans Serif Font is without feet. Sans Serif Fonts most often appear in headlines and short-format writing because they grab the reader's attention. A Sans Serif Font conveys modernity and lightness. It makes a short brand name pop. Top picks for Sans Serif Fonts include:

Helvetica

Optima

Futura

Think of the logo process as trying on hats. Once you find the right structure for your hat, you can begin to customize the shapes, colors, accents and other details. The goal for the design is to appeal to prospects rather than personal preference.

Now let's get into the design process. First, look back at the Message and Design Equation. Think about what you want to communicate visually that will convey what you have written. What shapes come to mind? What two or three colors? What objects come to mind? Consider common objects such as plants, animals, foods, letters and numbers that are universally recognizable and therefore memorable. Get creative, even so far as to become abstract. Once you think of a few objects that best represent the Message and Design Equation, ask yourself, "What is a new and different way to show this? Of those ways, which fit best with my equation?"

Sketch out on paper the ideas that come to mind. There is no bad idea at this point. Just put ideas down on paper. Afterward, sort out and select the strongest options. Circle the favorites. Cross off any that rank lower on the Message and Design Equation. Stick to the process. The logo options will be spot-on if they reflect your Message and Design Equation. They will feel right in your gut.

Present the strongest sketch ideas to two or three of your team members. Start by sharing with them the Message and Design Equation, and explain the logo must represent this equation. This is less a matter of opinion and more of a strategic process. Show them the proposed logos. Narrow it down to the two strongest ideas.

Now you have two logo semifinalists. Turn the sketches over to a graphic designer to create both logos for final consideration.

Or you can design them yourself. Start by scanning the sketches into a computer. At this stage, it is good to more fully explore different variations on font and color. Give both logos a color palette, preferably each a different one. Be sure the colors match the Message and Design Equation. Keep refining until you and the team feel like the logos are finished.

When you see the logo for the first time it will be alone on the page. The prospects typically see logos in the context of something bigger, as part of a website or a sign. Once you lock in the logo and colors, it will really come to life in your business card, mailer or other marketing tactics.

The last thing to do is print the two finished logos in large format, stand back and see which one feels best.

Choose your logo!

FLOURISH! logo development is no longer a mystery. It's a method.

ADDING A TAGLINE

Once the logo is complete, consider whether a tagline is needed.

The tagline is necessary when the organization name alone does not articulate what it does or its value offered. Think of it as a motto or a slogan to succinctly clarify the mission.

For example, the community name The Argyle is so basic it may require a tagline to demonstrate the value. The community's surveys revealed they are best known for encouraging happiness in residents, so they added the tagline, "Where happiness comes to life." This clarifies their value to inquiring residents and families.

The tagline is based upon the Message and Design Equation and answers the question: What does it do at what value? It provides excellent name recognition when it works. Think: Nothing Runs Like a Deere, Johnny on the Spot, Diamonds are Forever. A plumbing service in Kentucky boasts a clever poker analogy, "A Flush Beats A Full House."

A tagline isn't based on conjecture. It's based on the *FLOURISH!* method.

A TECHNIQUE FOR SIGNS

If signage is one of the tactics on your Balanced Marketing Formula, here is a technique for the sign design.

Begin by researching whether the landlord or property owner's association has any restrictions. Keep in mind any obstructions of view that will need to be overcome.

With those parameters in mind, consider where exterior signage is needed – perhaps on the exterior door, on the area above the entrance or on the outside wall of the building. Signage may need to appear in multiple areas. Consider as well where interior signage will be required – maybe way-finding signs in the building lobby, on an interior door or behind the front desk.

Negotiate price discounts with the signage installer when you order multiple signs at once.

Next, sketch on paper all that comes to mind pertaining to the signage. The logo will be the foundation. What else is needed? A tagline? Directional arrow? Lighting? Outdoor signage will need adequate lighting to be visible at night, and it will also need to be made of materials that will withstand the elements.

Refine the sketches. Select the stronger option to send to the sign company. Require that they send a proof of the sign before installation. Ask the vendor to Photoshop the mockup onto an image of the area where it will be installed. Ask for front and side views of the mockups to get a complete perspective.

Once you approve the mockups, the installer should provide final schematics and secure any required permits for installation. The only thing left is make sure signage is delivered and quality-checked.

Ta da! You have signs!

TOP 10 MISTAKES IN BRAND AWARENESS

1. **Being unimaginative.** Skip the standard font for the logo, like Arial or Times New Roman, in favor of getting creative with a custom or lesser-known font that best represents your organization.
2. **Jumping the gun.** Share logo or sign designs only after you have finalized them with the core team, but not while they are still under development.
3. **Stroking the ego.** As you proceed through logo and sign development, suspend the urge to design in your favorite color. Use instead colors and images that resonate with prospects.
4. **Defaulting to the obvious.** In logo or sign development, avoid using obvious objects like images of houses or stock icons. Experiment instead with objects that every person can relate to, prospects most importantly. Be creative.
5. **Cutting costs at all costs.** Online graphic design marketplaces are all the rage. They will design your logo for as little as $5. To have them design the logo or anything else without the *FLOURISH!* method would be unstrategic and therefore unreliable. Plus, you get what you pay for. Stick to the marketing budget.
6. **Sensational branding.** Resist the urge toward "sensational," or intentionally misspelled, branding. These include Blu-ray, Cheez-It and Dunkin' Donuts. Also known as "divergent" spelling, sensational spelling is not advised for aging services organizations for fear of trivializing the brand.

7. **Overdoing a good thing.** Many logos lose their power because their typeface is hard to read or muddled. There's a fine line between being clever and too cute. Aim for a logo that is memorable, simple and easy to read.

8. **Incomplete statement.** Together, an effective logo and a good tagline complete a sentence. They say what the organization does at what value to whom. If the logo doesn't make the whole statement, add a tagline.

9. **Expecting results.** Results from brand awareness tactics are tough to measure since they may not directly lead to new inquiries. Instead, measure results against the whole Balanced Marketing Formula.

10. **Not investing.** Brand awareness tactics go a long way in terms of demonstrating the organization's value to potential clients and families. Be sure to allot a portion of marketing budget to brand awareness for steady overall results from the Balanced Marketing Formula.

PART THREE

TRADITIONAL MEDIA

Traditional media has gotten a bum rap ever since the so-called Age of Empowerment arrived in advertising and marketing. Some aging services organizations are under the false impression that everything today is happening online, and they neglect to balance their marketing formula by including this critical strategy.

Almost all aging services organizations benefit from deploying a few tactics in traditional media. If brand awareness is about staying top-of-mind, then traditional media is about remaining front and center.

Consider the survey results to see which traditional media tactics are right for your organization. Do respondents remember seeing that last direct mail piece from your organization? Do they pay attention to billboards around town? Do they read the local newspaper or city magazine? Do they have a favorite radio or television station?

Recall the allotment of marketing budget you assigned to traditional media. A common misperception holds that traditional media are expensive or have low returns compared to online marketing. In fact, a direct mail campaign can lead to an immediate spike in new inquiries precisely when needed, and that sends revenue to the bottom line. Return to the foundation you set for the *FLOURISH!* method to create the traditional media mix that will work best.

Media buys are often negotiated and discounted for volume. When you get ready to purchase, ask the account representative for the rate sheet, which will show the cost of the media reduced over the number of times it runs. The longer the run, the lower the rate.

Sometimes one rep can purchase media for you across a variety of media such as billboards and radio all in one.

Be sure to ask if they offer online marketing to complement your traditional media tactics. Some newspaper reps, for example, will run your ad in the print or web editions at no additional cost.

Part Three will explore how to get the most out of traditional media with the four tactics of direct mail, print advertising, billboard advertising and broadcast advertising.

DIRECT MAIL DEBUNKED

The first indication that your organization can benefit from direct mail is that the surveys validated it has worked in the past.

Direct mail works great if competition is fierce and you need to secure an initial foothold in the market. It positions your organization as a resource of genuine value to your area by programming the immediate surrounding population to think of you first above others and to perceive you a certain way.

Direct mail can be a hefty investment, but it can really pay off. That said, this tactic is best outsourced to an expert.

Direct mail supports the health and lifespan of the organization by injecting a steady shot of advertising each time a mailer "drops," or is mailed out. This tactic is great for organizations that need an immediate boost in new inquiries and especially for new aging services organizations.

Keep in mind, each spike is followed by a dip. That's why it's important to embrace repetition and to supplement direct mail with the other tactics in the Balanced Marketing Formula.

When developing a direct mail campaign, first qualify and quantify your market. Define the target market by articulating what the ideal direct mail recipients might have in common: affluent retirees, $100,000 income, recently bought a boat. The more granular the picture, the better focused the campaign.

A reputable direct mail agency will overlay the attributes of the target audience with data from demographic reports to attract just the right prospects.

Have a look at the marketing budget, and share with the direct mail vendor the amount allotted to this tactic. Confine the vendor to an effective campaign within that budget.

Be sure to agree on the goal and quantify how many new inquiries are needed from the campaign to achieve the desired return on investment.

Before pulling the trigger, ask how the vendor will identify results. A custom phone number can track which new inquiries originated from which mailer. The vendor should report after each drop a breakdown of how many households were hit.

Particularly in this marketing tactic, it is critical to stick to the Message and Design Equation. The value and offer have to be crystal clear or the effort is fruitless. And don't try to cram ten pounds of text into a five-pound mailer.

A direct mail vendor can guide your team through the creative process to develop the most effective campaign for the organization. Direct mail experts have a specific formula for crafting the right pieces within any given campaign. Moreover, they design each piece to keep the eye moving to all the critical areas in just a few seconds. All of this drives results by making a compelling offer. The specific formula creates a high level of interest. The mailer should not divulge all the information at once, but instead motivate the reader to take the next step.

A direct mail piece is dead in the water without an offer. Without some incentive, the prospect is left hanging. The offer is nothing more than a motivator to get the reader to take action.

In formulating the offer, bear in mind that discounts in direct mail tend to turn the organization into a commodity and can diminish perceived value. The offer doesn't have to include a discount, but it does need to be valuable to the prospect. Offering a complimentary tour, for example, is not discounting your services. Rather, it's opening a door.

Be sure the phone number is large and legible on the direct mailer. That's likely the next logical step they will take – call for more information.

Use this as a guide for working with the right direct mail vendor and you will get more new inquiries from this tactic.

When backed by the *FLOURISH!* method, direct mail can work wonders.

PRINT ADVERTISING STRATEGY

Print advertising may surface in your Balanced Marketing Formula. Perhaps this is because the surveys show clients and families are avid readers of the local newspaper or a particular magazine. Or perhaps you have tested print advertising in the past and determined that it delivers a strong return on investment.

The best print ads tell a story. The object is not to inform ad nauseam, but to inspire. Keep reminding yourself and your team that no one can tell your organization's story like your happiest clients and families. Create a print ad campaign that features testimonials and real stories from clients and their families. You might even draw upon the survey results to craft these stories. (Be sure to execute a signed release form for HIPAA compliance.)

A strong print ad has a short, eye-catching headline. As mentioned in The Science Behind the Logo in Part Two, a Sans Serif Font is more legible for quick reading.

Avoid using the organization's name or logo as the head-line. That would be like walking into a crowded room and announcing, "We are Grafton Senior Living!" Instead, use a clever phrase to draw the reader's attention. Once you pique interest, the reader will find the name and contact details, toward the bottom of the ad design.

People are visual creatures. Lighten up on the text and go big with an appealing and relevant graphic. Avoid stock photography in favor of custom professional shots of the care team and clients. Again, be sure to get a signed model release form. Go with what will be inviting to the prospect, not necessarily your favorite shots.

Be sure to use high-resolution photography. The term "resolution" refers to the detail in an image. The greater the detail, the more crisply it will reproduce in print. Low-resolution photos are fine for use on the web, but print always requires high-resolution imagery.

The best ads provide an "a-ha!" moment, or get a chuckle. Get creative and include a clever and memorable twist to your ad. If you're really feeling bold, ask the publication to run it upside down, and include a small disclaimer at the bottom – or in this case, top – saying "Intentionally run upside down." Use a popular phrase to rope in readers. "Leaks Like a Sieve" was the headline for a roofing company ad that ran for a long time, and while I haven't seen the ad in years, I still remember it because it made me smile.

Be sure to include a compelling call-to-action. This is the equivalent of the direct mail offer. Incentivize the reader to take the next step: Free tour. New-resident gift. Complimentary consultation. Then tell the reader exactly how to take the next step: Call today. Make an appointment. Email for more information.

Be sure that clear contact information appears in the ad. At the very least, include the phone number and web address.

As with all traditional media, consistency is key. Run the same campaign at least 10 times in the same publication to be noticed, and even longer to be remembered. With a dynamic print ad strategy backed by the *FLOURISH!* method, new inquiries will be consistent rather than erratically swinging up and down over time.

BLUEPRINT FOR BILLBOARDS

Billboard advertising is likely in your Balanced Marketing Formula if the surveys validated this tactic, and if you aim to reach a vast and diverse population across a certain geographic area.

Advertising on multiple billboards around town typically achieves the greatest reach. This marketing tactic can require a significant investment. Be sure it's what's best for reaching your goals. Under the right circumstances, it can be a good way to regularly attract a large number of new inquiries.

Billboards work best when they run in conjunction with other traditional media efforts. The message on the billboard has to match the one running in the city magazine ads, which matches the jingle playing every Tuesday morning on the radio during rush hour. It all ties together.

Billboards are not just signs along the highway. Many city centers feature brightly illuminated digital billboards that were first made popular in Times Square. Large-format advertising on the side of city buses and metro rail systems may gain more attention than their stationary counterparts. Seniors appreciate big type.

Pith is the essence of billboard messaging. You have only a split second to grab the eye and share one concept. Sukle, an advertising agency in Denver, nailed pith and brevity with their billboards for Denver Water. The campaign was so clever that the trade journal AdWeek featured it as exemplary. Read more about it at www.adweek.com/topic/denver-water.

The anatomy of a billboard that drives results is simple: Headline, no more than 12 words, followed by logo. That's it. You don't even have to include the phone number or website. If the billboard is catchy enough, people will search you out from the name in the logo.

Billboards for healthcare organizations can indeed be humorous. Here's one for a hospital under construction: "Keep your eyes on the road, we are not open yet."

Short format is the most difficult to write. As Mark Twain famously put it, "I didn't have time to write a shorter letter." To write a catchy billboard, make it a game with your team to come up with clever, funny or catchy phrases of 12 words or fewer that tie back to your Message and Design Equation.

Eventually the winners will emerge and your billboard campaign will be launched. And any billboard campaign grounded in the *FLOURISH!* method will yield more regular results.

FOOLPROOF BROADCAST ADVERTISING

Perhaps it was revealed on the surveys that broadcast advertising, such as television and radio ads, should appear in your Balanced Marketing Formula.

Broadcast ads work very well in tandem with billboards to provide wide-reaching awareness across a particular geographic region. Like billboard advertising, television and radio ads require a significant investment, so be sure to budget wisely. When done right, these ads pack the power to attract a multitude of new inquiries, so the returns can be quite robust.

Writing and producing television and radio ads is complicated, so it's best left to media experts. With this type of traditional media, the media rep placing the ad may be able to oversee writing the ad copy and having the spot recorded with professional voiceover and actors. Be sure to ask.

A television or radio commercial is often referred to as a "spot." Hold the rep accountable for creating a top-notch spot for you with specific guidelines:

1. Begin by sharing your Messaging and Design Equation with the media rep.
2. Ask to see the script before the spot is produced, and be sure that the writing reflects your Messaging and Design Equation. Humor works very well in broadcast advertising, but only if it fits your organization. Emotional appeals can also work well, but shy away from fear-based advertis-

ing as it doesn't produce results as well as positive ads do.

3. As with other traditional media, the offer is key. Make sure the offer and contact information are clearly articulated. In broadcast advertising, it can be advantageous to have the contact information repeated several times in the spot for easy recall. Listeners or viewers often have mobile devices in hand while consuming the broadcast message. There's no better time to get them to act than right now.

4. A vanity phone number or memorable website address goes a long way in broadcast advertising. Caring Senior Service uses 1-800-SENIOR-CARE.

5. A jingle, including the organization's name and phone number, can also help with recall. A jingle works best when the name is short and easy to sing. Be sure to use the same jingle for every ad. Consistency is key when tapping recall.

6. Use the same voiceover or acting talent for added memorability. For years, Allison Janney was the voice behind every one of Kaiser Permanente's broadcast ads, both television and radio. TMZ describes her voice as "so soothing that it can make even the worst of news seem okay."

7. After the ad is scripted, the media rep will get it recorded or produced. Review the final ad with three Ds in mind: distinctive, digestible, deed-oriented. It is distinctive when it reflects your Messaging and Design Equation and sets you apart from the competition. It is digestible when it tells one cohesive story that is easy to understand and clearly articulated. It is deed-oriented when it asks the listener or viewer act, to take the next step and extends an offer to inspire them to do so.

8. As with print and billboard advertising, extended campaigns work better than a single ad. Once the media company develops the first great ad, have them expand it into at least a three-part series. A campaign tells a bigger story and gains greater brand awareness.

You can have faith in your broadcast advertising approach knowing that it's anchored in the *FLOURISH!* method.

TOP 10 MISTAKES IN TRADITIONAL MEDIA

1. **Ignoring traditional media.** Resist the notion that traditional media is passé. Most aging services organizations can benefit from investing some portion of the marketing budget into these tactics to stay front and center.

2. **One and done.** Avoid the urge to run one advertisement or mail a single postcard. Generally speaking, a prospect has to read/see/hear an offer ten times for it even to be noticed, let alone acted upon. Repetition is key to all traditional media. Even better, repetition across traditional media tactics can propel the organization to ubiquity. Besides, campaigns are always more successful than single efforts. How many times did you see the promo for a television show before you tuned in?

3. **Confusing informative with persuasive.** The goal is to get the reader to take the next step, not give all of the details at once. This goes not just for direct mail, but also for print and billboard advertising as well as broadcast advertising.

4. **Faking it.** Real photos will best sell the story. Forego stock photography in favor of custom professional shots of the care team and clients, securing a signed model release for HIPAA compliance.

5. **Trifold brochures.** The standard trifold brochure is dated. Instead, invest in a welcome packet. It's like the sexy booklet that car dealers give out when you take a test drive. The welcome packet is engaging and sharable. It gives prospects the feeling, "Wow, I belong here!" and offers

family members peace of mind.

6. **Sponsorships.** Everywhere you turn, aging services organizations are asked to sponsor something. "Exhibit right alongside all of your competitors at the area senior care event… Buy a booth at the local 5K run… Participate in the neighborhood co-op door-to-door flyer that includes the logo of every business in the area." Your organization will get lost in the clutter. It's always good to give back, so strategically select only one or two sponsorships for the year. Advertising dollars are better spent on direct marketing and high-visibility awareness than these limited-impact initiatives.

7. **Long format.** Brevity and clarity trump long format in traditional media. Keep text short and simple.

8. **Low-balling on identity.** Be sure to invest in well-designed business cards, letterhead and envelopes – otherwise known as identity. These traditional marketing tactics speak volumes about brand reputation. A heavy card stock communicates trustworthiness, for example.

9. **Stopping short.** Radio and television ads should be repurposed on the website and social media pages. This stuff is online gold. Web users love little sound bites and short videos. Plus, the better the ads, the more apt they are to be shared.

10. **Failure to proof.** Once traditional media hits the streets, there's no turning back. An ad in Houston hit 500,000 households reading ABORTION ATTORNEY instead of adoption attorney. If a mistake or typo leaks out there, it's nowhere near as easy or inexpensive to correct as with online efforts. Be sure to proofread the ad copy carefully.

PART FOUR

ONLINE PROMOTION

Online promotion is all the rage. Facebook, Twitter, Insta-gram, Google, Bing, Yahoo! – they are fun to say, they are hot and a lot of aging services organizations are all over them.

Why?

We are a gadget-obsessed culture, and there is no greater gadget than the World Wide Web. The web is the only form of media that gives us so much individual control. You can become a published blogger overnight. Order that new book online right now and start reading it on your tablet immedi-ately. Amazon Prime Air will soon deliver wares in 30 minutes or less, like a pizza, via drone rather than driver. Hired a new employee? No problem. Just log onto the website and upload her photo and bio. Instant gratification never felt so right.

Plus, there is a lingering belief that online promotion is far less expensive than traditional media. In the early days, online promotion was commonly thought of as free. Just jump online, post your information and get instant exposure in front of prospects.

If only it were that easy.

A Balanced Marketing Formula includes online promotion among other strategies. It can be easy to get carried away with the online craze by overinvesting. There are so many online promotion options available that it's easy to bite off too much. The Balanced Marketing Formula keeps you on track and on budget.

Be sure that the marketing budget allots an appropriate percentage to online promotions. Not too high, not too low – refer to the Balanced Marketing Formula at the end of Part One to be sure of the right investment. Go back to the survey results to understand which online promotions to focus on. What do people like about the website, and what needs improvement? Are prospects searching online for their senior care needs? Are potential clients and families frequenting Facebook, or do they prefer Instagram?

Part Four shows how to get the most out of online promotions, including website, social media, search exposure and reputation management.

DISCIPLINED WEBSITE DESIGN

Suppose the surveys indicated your organization's website needs a makeover.

Keep it simple. A 15-page website is adequate for a small to mid-sized aging services organization, even one with multiple locations. One of those pages can be dedicated to the blog, which will fill in with entries over time and enhance the content of the website. Like marketing on the whole, the website is a living organism. Rich, relevant content and frequent updates are what make a website visible on search engines. But beware of content overdose. Quality trumps quantity.

If you bristled at the word "blog" thinking it is a huge undertaking, fear not. Think of the blog as nothing more than an online journal. Excerpts of published articles, conversations with other senior care professionals and muses on your team's care all make interesting and easy-to-formulate fodder. Don't carry the weight alone. Some of the entries can come from your own team's writings. Then pick up other sources to round it out. Search online for expert material that can be reposted (and be sure it's properly credited). Have staff write guest blog entries about what it's like to work there. Invite a resident to describe what it's like to be under your care, transcribing the story to post to the blog. (Be sure to get a HIPAA compliant release.) Post once a week and the blog will grow over time.

Be sure the website provides an "action opportunity" on every page. "Call for a tour... Fill out a form to learn more... Follow us on Facebook... Enter an email address and get a free care guide." Each person who arrives at the website will have different preferences, so provide a number of options. The more options, the more likely web visitors are to act and thereby stay engaged.

The website should be designed to whet the appetite and encourage action. Be sure that the web text and look matches your Message and Design Equation and is promotional rather than informational.

Stick to the three A's of websites that drive results: affability, ability, availability.

A powerful website makes the organization look affable, or likable. Visitors should see warm and inviting photos of the organization, team and clients, with HIPAA compliant releases completed. Visitors should get the feeling, "I might like them. They could earn my trust."

A great website makes it readily evident that the staff is highly able. Any of the team's awards and accolades and any compelling stories of client happiness and success should be evident in the first few seconds of looking at the home page. Visitors should get the feeling, "They seem capable. They would take good care of me."

A terrific website articulates the senior care team is available. Clear contact information for all levels of care should appear on every page. This conveys the feeling, "It would be easy for me to at least check them out. I could make it happen."

Website development is a lot like building a home: it's a big process and a huge investment; it opens up high probability of scope, time and budget creep; and, the finished product is a public reflection of you and your organization, which means it has to be just right.

Use eight proven milestones to guide your provider to completion:

1. **Budget.** Share with the web developer the budget you have allocated, and execute a written agreement stipulating those terms.
2. **Sitemap.** This is the blueprint for the website. The web developer should outline in text the navigation of the site, demonstrate the page flow and show the titles of all pages. Be sure that your team and theirs fully agree on the sitemap before proceeding. After the blueprint is approved, construction begins. Adding a room on a house later (or adding a webpage) can drive up costs and compromise the integrity of the original design.
3. **Web Text.** Request that your provider write, edit and proofread all text to appear on the website. Share your Message and Design Equation to eliminate the guesswork and streamline the process. Be sure to lock in the web text before going to the next step. Just as a bathroom with one sink has a different configuration than a bathroom with two, webpages similarly shift with more or less text.
4. **Wireframe.** Ask for a basic layout of the functionality of the website. Will there be a large "slider" of compelling images on the home page? Where will images appear, and where will text appear? Where will action opportunities appear? Be sure to see a wireframe for the home page and at least one other page. This part of the process is like the newly framed home. You and your team will begin to see what it will be like when it's finished. Refine and sign off on the wireframe to go to the most exciting part: the actual build-out.

5. **Homepage Design.** Focus on the homepage first. This way, you can see the heart of the house nearly finished before the other rooms are designed. As with everything else, be sure the homepage design correlates with your organization's Message and Design Equation. Approving this will set the rest of the build out in motion.

6. **Website Development.** The rest of the webpages should be developed from the foundation set in steps 2 through 5. A great deal of sophisticated computer coding may be required. This may be a good step to outsource to an expert if you haven't already used an outside agency in the previous steps. The foundation locks in the direction for the rest of the design, making the development process much faster and more exciting. Rather than build a separate mobile site, which was a popular solution in the early 2010s, have your provider build the website to be "responsive." This means the website will automatically resize to various screen sizes (phone, tablet, laptop, desktop). The content will be responsive regardless of where it appears.

7. **Testing.** Prior to launch, be sure functionality is tested across all browsers and devices to ensure quality display regardless of who's viewing it where.

8. **Launch!**

The website is a billboard in the middle of the ocean until you make the effort to attract visitors with tactics like social media, search engine optimization (SEO) and online advertising. These are the tactics that transform the website into an efficient machine that attracts visitors to your site and inquiries to your door while your team focuses on what they do best: serving older adults. That's the *FLOURISH!* method for you.

DEMYSTIFYING SOCIAL MEDIA

"We don't have a choice on whether we do social media," warns Erik Qualman, author of *Socialnomics*. "The question is how well we do it."

In his YouTube video of the same title, he points out:

- 90% of buying decisions are influenced by social media
- By 2018, video will account for two-thirds of mobile usage
- 1 in 3 marriages start online
- Every second, 2 people join LinkedIn
- The fastest growing demographic on Twitter is grandparents

While Qualman makes a good point that social media can't be ignored, it's not that scary. In fact, social media is nothing more than an open house. It's just happening online.

Here are several guidelines from the book *Social Media is a Cocktail Party*, by Jim Tobin and Lisa Braziel:

- **"The event goes on with or without you."** Whether or not you are participating, people are talking about your organization online. Why not join the conversation?
- **"Listen and mingle before you talk."** You wouldn't want to monopolize the conversation offline, so be careful not to do so online either.

- **"Different settings have different rules of etiquette."** Just as you would behave differently at a children's birthday party than you would at a business networking lunch, Facebook requires a different decorum than LinkedIn. If Facebook is like an open house, then LinkedIn is the gathering of collaborating aging services professionals.
- **"You can ask for a little help from your friends."** Once you build a base of followers who love your organization, they will write stellar reviews and refer more often. After all, anything for a friend.
- **"Share information that doesn't benefit you."** Apply the 80/20 rule. Be promotional 20% of the time, and talk about other things of interest to your following the rest of the time.
- **"Make it about them, not about you."** People love to talk about themselves. Let them. When it's your turn, they will be all ears.

Let's dive deeper into best practices for Facebook. Post at least two to three times a week to stay visible. Anytime your organization's page gets a comment on a post, have someone on staff comment back as soon as possible to keep the conversation going.

Make it possible for others to post on your organization's page. (Adjust this on the privacy settings.) Inviting others to post on your page opens the door to your open house and invites others to be part of it.

Finally, invite people to like your page. Include a "Like Us on Facebook" link in team email signatures, on the website – everywhere. Run a Facebook ad to get even more likes. Facebook ads are explored in the next section.

Now for LinkedIn best practices. First, be sure everyone on your team has an updated profile page. Prospects and referrers will likely look for you and your teammates online before calling or committing; therefore, complete and relevant profiles are mandatory. Don't make profiles a cut-and-paste of resumes. Instead, train the staff to draw readers into their profiles with elements from the organization's Message and Design Equation.

Make the profiles public by adjusting settings. The more people who see you and your team, the more new inquiries and referrals you will attract.

Recommend others on LinkedIn. Don't just make endorsements by clicking on the buttons on people's profiles. Take the time to write a short but detailed review about what they did for your organization and how it helped. Over time, many will do the same for you, and these reviews act as online referrals. You can't beat word-of-mouth.

For more exposure on LinkedIn, get involved in groups and discussion boards. Repurpose blog postings to stay relevant and visible in multiple conversations. Whenever someone comments on a post, be sure to respond to keep the conversation going.

Let's talk about virality (not to be confused with virility). Virality is the tendency to spread by word of mouth. It's all about cracking the code on getting noticed on social media. Posts that get high virality, or are liked, commented on, and shared most often are: photos of the team, babies or dogs (or better yet, babies with dogs), happy birthday posts (and also happy wedding or happy new baby) and funny images or cartoons. Think of things that will make people smile.

Posts that get low virality include polls and questions that require too much thinking and long posts that require too much reading. This is a social setting, not a seminar. No one likes the overt intellectual or long-winded talker to overtake the conversation. Keep it light.

Social media can be a slippery slope in this open-communications era. Never post anything that may violate HIPAA privacy regulations. Train all staff members who are posting on social media to follow common-sense guidelines:

1. If you wouldn't say it in an elevator, don't say it online.
2. Don't post about clients, even in general terms, unless there is a signed consent form on file.
3. Do post about situations, solutions and research relevant to senior care.
4. Don't badmouth the competition, even subtly.
5. Do use humor carefully.
6. When in doubt, leave it out.

Abe was right: It's impossible to please all of the people all of the time. Inevitably, you will get a negative social media post or comment. When it happens, behave just like you would with a disgruntled family member acting out for all to see. Respond publicly. Use a simple reply like, "Thank you for your feedback. We will do everything we can to rectify the situation." Then call them. Be calm and understanding, listening intently until all emotion about the issue has been exhausted. If a resolution is reached, consider asking the person to remove the post.

Above all else, take the high road in social media. Behave with the ultimate decorum, and it will reflect favorably on your organization.

Social media is only one tactic in the Balanced Marketing Formula. Avoid the temptation to get too carried away overinvesting time or thought to it. Use the *FLOURISH!* method, and your team will be able to stay the course for steady results.

A SYSTEM FOR ATTRACTING WEB VISITORS

The right tactics for attracting web visitors surface in nearly every aging services organization's Balanced Marketing Formula. It's a matter of figuring out which tactics are best to deploy at any given time. There are so many tactics that even savvy marketers can get overwhelmed.

As always, first consider the survey results. Would existing clients and families search online for an organization like yours? Would they click on the ads, or only the organic search results? Would they follow your organization on Facebook? Eliminate irrelevant tactics from the list.

Consider the funnel on the following page, the brainchild of Ryan Wilson of FiveFifty Digital Marketing, to further simplify the possibilities.

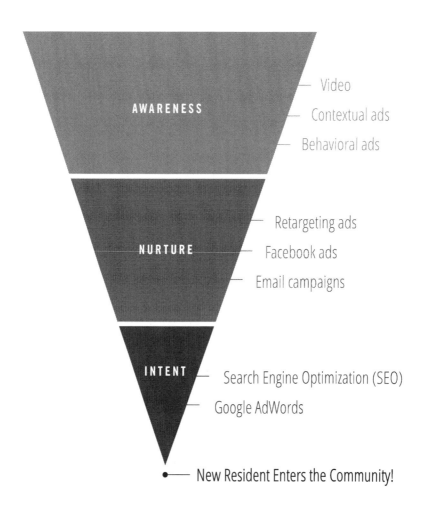

Awareness

The top and largest section of Wilson's funnel is awareness. For new aging services organizations, the immediate goal is to increase awareness of offerings. No one knows about the organization yet, but they will soon with tactics of video, contextual ads and behavioral ads.

A video makes most sense when it can be repurposed across several media. For example, a television spot can be added to the website homepage and shared across social media for maximum exposure.

Like retargeting ads, contextual and behavioral ads are colorfully designed, sometimes animated or flashy ads. Contextual ads appear on websites that have a context closely linked to the organization's offering. Behavioral ads appear on websites that match the online profile (or behavior) of those most likely to become clients, or their families.

The experts typically best handle all awareness tactics. It's a big investment, but it pays off over time.

In 2007 GoDaddy.com invested millions of dollars in Super Bowl ads that subsequently went viral online. While they didn't capture an immediate monetary return on investment, they reportedly drew 1.5 million visits to the GoDaddy.com website. Suddenly everyone knew GoDaddy.com. This is top-of-mind awareness at its finest. After that game, whenever someone was ready to buy a website address, GoDaddy.com was the place to go.

***

Nurture

Consider the next concept in Wilson's funnel: the pool of potential clients and families that can be nurtured into the organization. These are people who may have a need in the future or who have made initial contact but not yet taken the next action. While they may not be ready to take that next step today, they are likely to in the next six months.

Nurture tactics help the organization show up in the right place at the right time. They most often include retargeting ads, Facebook ads, Facebook promoted posts and email campaigns.

Retargeting ads include more than just text like Google AdWords. Often called banner ads, they are colorfully designed, sometimes animated or flashy visuals that follow people around the web. Let's say a potential resident or family member visits your website but wanders off to other sites. A banner ad can appear atop multiple pages on those other sites to keep the organization top-of-mind.

Facebook ads work similarly, appearing in the newsfeeds of people who are likely to someday visit the organization. This visibility nurtures the potential resident and family to think of you when the time is right. Facebook's promoted posts make it possible to plug the fact that certain people like your page and may invite other like-minded folks to do the same.

Daily posting on the organization's Facebook page is the unpaid way to capture this mindshare and can boost top-of-mind awareness.

As with SEO and Google AdWords, a one-two punch can pack a bigger bang. Retargeting ads, Facebook ads and Facebook promoted posts are best handled by the experts. Email campaigns are a great do-it-yourself option to nurture prospects to take the next step. Push it beyond the typical business newsletter. Create a series of emails that reflect your Message and Design Equation. Consider repurposing direct mail or print/billboard advertising campaigns into this digital medium for maximum effect.

***

Intent
Refer back to Wilson's funnel at the beginning of this section. The bottom and smallest area is packed full of people who seek an organization like yours. It's easier and cheaper to reach the people who already have intent to find an aging services organization like yours. "Right this very moment there are potential clients who already need your services," explains Wilson. "It's just a matter of helping them find *you*."

These are the folks who reside in the intent section of the funnel: they understand that they have a senior care need, they know they have to seek out a solution and they are ready to take the next action once they find the right provider. This is the low-hanging fruit. It's comparatively inexpensive to get intentional people to take those steps of calling or signing an agreement.

Intent tactics typically include SEO and Google AdWords. There is a big difference between the two:

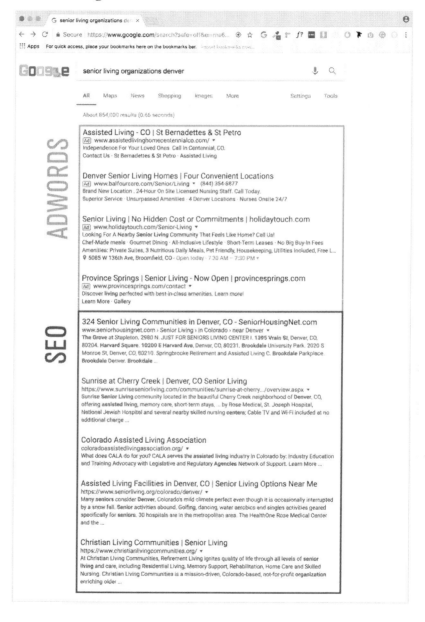

SEO drives websites to the top of the "organic" listings through methods of enriching website content. Google, Yahoo! and Bing crawl the web continuously to search out the most robust websites and present them as top choices for the searched keywords. A search strategist will keep your organization's name highly visible on search engines by keeping the website healthy and active with relevant content, working links and a variety of other goodies that search engines hunt.

SEO used to be a simple process of stuffing keywords into a website and bolstering website headings with highly searched terms. Today it is a far more complex strategy. On average, Google changes its search algorithm 1.37 times every *day*. That means search strategists have to continuously stay on the leading edge to keep the organization's website on page one of the search results.

The more relevant the content and the more regular updates the website has, the more robust it appears to the search engines, and the higher it climbs in the search results. SEO is like car maintenance – the tasks for upkeep continue over the lifetime of the vehicle.

Google AdWords is simply an online auction. Competing aging services organizations essentially outbid each other so their online ad shows most often. Each keyword, such as "Austin assisted living," is given a dollar value, and the highest bidder's ad shows up first atop the page. The charge is triggered not when the ad shows but when someone clicks on the ad. Hence, the term pay-per-click advertising. This is where Google makes its millions, by making it easy for organizations to set up and manage their own campaigns.

Easy to set up and manage, sure. But it's more complicated to create a campaign that will drive results. A good search strategist will help select highly searched words and terms at a reasonable cost that are most likely to convert clicks into inquiries. A good ad leads not just to the website homepage but to a relevant *landing page* that echoes the offer in the ad. The landing page increases the likelihood that the prospect will take the next step: call, or take a tour for example. Like any good ad, AdWords can get the resident and family in the door. The rest is up to your team, which requires having a dynamic website and a solid new resident admission process.

It doesn't matter whether you or your teammates are more apt to stick to the organic search results or to click the ads on the Google results. It matters only how your prospects behave online.

SEO and Google AdWords are not do-it-yourself tactics. Lean on a strong search strategist to get the most out of your investment. Combining both can more quickly drive new inquiries.

✳✳✳

Each part of the funnel feeds into the next. Wilson advises, "If you have strong website traffic but visitors are not filling out the online form or calling in, that indicates the need to move people from nurture to intent. If your website traffic is low, that indicates a need for more awareness."

Some organizations benefit from regularly running one or two tactics in each area of the funnel. Many simply stick to nurture tactics to maintain the status quo of new inquiries through top-of-mind awareness. All healthy organizations keep coming back to the Balanced Marketing Formula to ensure a good spread of strategies, both online and offline.

The great thing about online efforts is that they are highly measurable. Be sure to set up Google Analytics to track website traffic. Gather monthly reporting on online marketing efforts. Consider these reports like you would financial investment statements: look for overall trends but try not to get too caught up in the details.

With online promotion, so much of the decision happens before the lead even contacts the organization. Work the funnel with the guidelines provided here, and you will have applied the fruitful *FLOURISH!* method to the organization's online marketing strategy, too.

REPUTATION MANAGEMENT SIMPLIFIED

Reputation management is public relations on the web – it's all about keeping your organization's reputation squeaky clean.

Hired specialists scour the web to uncover reviews and other content that may be damaging to the brand name. Some reputation management services help cover up bad reviews by stuffing the web with good reviews or other content. This essentially pushes negative reviews further down in search results.

Be proactive rather than reactive. The more aware you are, the better positioned you are to immediately respond to marginal reviews. There are three things you can do today:

First, set up a Google Alert with your organization's name to receive regular updates about what's appearing on the web bearing the brand name.

Second, get social. The more active your organization is online, the more apt you are to get positive reviews and to see negative reviews as they happen.

Third, take quick action on a bad review. Rule of thumb: Behave the same way you would if a resident or family member voiced a negative opinion within earshot of others. Always respond. To say nothing might convey arrogance or ambivalence, implying agreement with the criticism. Type up a professional response and review it with another team member for objectivity and clarity before posting. Depending upon the protocols of your organization, you may need to review it with the legal department. Afterward, call the complainant to hear his side of the story and offer a resolution.

By the way, an overall rating of four stars is great on a scale of five. Five-star reviews across the board suggest review stuffing, or "astroturfing," which undermines credibility.

Reputation is built every day in every way. When your organization is humming along at its best, it will be reflected online just as it is in offline circles. In this way, the *FLOURISH!* method simplifies reputation management so you and your team can focus on care.

TOP 10 MISTAKES IN ONLINE PROMOTION

1. **Believing slick salespeople.** There are no guarantees in online promotion. Walk away from anything that sounds too good to be true. "We will get you found on page one of Google tomorrow…"

2. **Same old site.** There are a lot of cookie-cutter templates out there, but you don't want to look like the aging services organization next door. At the same time, there's no need to hassle with an expensive custom website. A happy medium is a customizable WordPress theme. Pick a theme and add your own design and content to stand out from the competition.

3. **Overdoing it.** In most cases, a 15-page website plus blog is plenty.

4. **Bad shots.** Use crisp, clear images of the organization and team (and with HIPAA compliant model release forms) in lieu of cliché stock photos.

5. **Confusing navigation.** To keep the potential resident or family member moving through the website and eventually to your online door, narrow down the navigation to no more than seven pages or "rails" across the top and no more than five on each dropdown. Group similar information on each page so the layout is digestible and well organized.

6. **Missing the opportunity.** Be sure the phone number, email address and links to the social media pages appear prominently on every web page. Better yet, include a short form on every page with an engaging offer: "Share your email address and get our article, '10 Questions to Ask

Before Moving Your Loved One into a Senior Care Community.'"

7. **Missing the party.** People are talking about your organization online. Join the conversation.

8. **DIY on the cheap.** Let go of the idea that a do-it-yourself solution for attracting website visitors will save money, and invest instead in a dedicated expert on your team or with an agency that can guide you through these tactics. It will pay off.

9. **Billboard at sea.** The website is a billboard in the middle of the ocean until you make the effort to attract visitors. Start with intent tactics first (SEO and Google AdWords), since they are the easiest and least expensive way to attract people who already have the intention of finding a an aging services organization like yours.

10. **Reputation management run amok.** Instead of worrying about bad reviews, focus on attracting great reviews by training your team to always be at its best.

PART FIVE

INTERNAL MARKETING

Internal marketing is the least expensive, most powerful and most *neglected* strategy.

What is internal marketing? It is a virtuous circle in which happy employees cultivate happy clients and families who attract more like-minded prospects. In other words, it is the ultimate employee retention, customer satisfaction and word-of-mouth marketing strategy. It becomes self-reinforcing and self-fulfilling.

Aging services organizations often extend special offers only to *new* clients and families. Smart organizations give special treatment to *current* clients and families, who are already loyal and have the power to bring more happy clients. And the smartest organizations give extra-special treatment to their employees, who are the most powerful people in the word-of-mouth marketing game.

It's easier and more cost-effective to cultivate a referred resident into a move-in than it is to transition a cold lead that comes from brand awareness, traditional marketing or online promotion. A referral is likely to need less education, have a shorter learning curve and bring stronger loyalty than a cold lead from other sources.

It is critical to *systematize* internal marketing. There are five steps:

1. Create a world-class culture
2. Hire right in the first place
3. Put employees first
4. Ratchet up the "ask" for referrals
5. Powerfully align sales with marketing

Internal marketing starts with motivated team members who are in the right environment and have a high level of job satisfaction – that's steps 1 through 3. Internal marketing requires team members who understand the organization's mission, vision and values. These team members are fiercely committed to reaching the organization's goals and have tangible personal goals closely tied with organizational growth. They are committed to delivering a high level of service and quality in every interaction.

Notice that the team comes before the clients. Happy team equals happy clients and families. You can't have the latter without the former.

Read on to find out exactly how to seamlessly take all five steps with the *FLOURISH!* method.

CREATE A WORLD-CLASS CULTURE

Organizational culture is made up of the mission, vision, values, goals, beliefs, attitudes and behaviors that all employees have in common. An aging services organization has a culture regardless if it has been strategically developed. The culture determines how employees relate to their work, to the organization at large and to the clients and families.

The surveys will reveal what the team thinks about the organization, what's appealing about working there and what's not. Look back for what the team shared in the surveys, which can easily springboard into the creation of mission, vision and values.

The *mission* answers this question: What is the organization's main purpose? It's why you and your team show up to work every day. It's very likely tied to your Message and Design Equation. For example, Applewood Our House's mission is, "To create new memories for our residents and families while treating each person as an individual who deserves respect and dignity while receiving outstanding and passionate care."

The *vision* is much larger and answers a key question: How does the organization envision changing the world? A vision statement might start with the phrase, "We imagine a world where..." For example, "We imagine a world where all older adults get the respect, dignity and care that they deserve." The vision makes the mission a global quest, beyond the walls of the organization.

The *values* answer this question: What is the organization's core ideology? Values are the basic beliefs that all team members have in common. Here's an example of a values statement, from Applewood Our House:

- We do what's right even when there is no one watching.
- We are considerate of others and their feelings; co-workers, residents and their families, our friends and loved ones.
- We show up to life on time and give it our all.
- We are open to other points of view.
- When our integrity grows, so does the trust that others place in us.

The nuances of how the mission, vision and values permeate into daily operations are endless. *How the phone is answered. Whether team members are smiling. What it says about a senior living community when a resident sits alone.*

Internal marketing circles back to brand. It's all about perception and experience. When employees make a resident and family a promise and the organization delivers on that promise, the clients and families have an excellent experience. Customers who have excellent experiences keep like-minded customers crossing the threshold.

Share the mission, vision and values with your team on a regular basis and in meaningful ways. Celebrate the small ways that employees represent mission, vision and values with Employee of the Month or even Moment of the Day.

Share with employees the organization's quantifiable goals. Perhaps it's to increase occupancy from 80% to 90% in three months. Or to improve the Star Quality Rating by one star in the next 12 months.

Or to open the financial books so that all employees understand the income, cost of goods, expenses and profits. Then work together to create a quantifiable goal to improve one or more of those areas. (You might be surprised how many 21st Century companies are doing this with great success.)

Next, have managers work one-on-one with each direct report to create an individual development plan (IDP). The IDP connects the organization's quantifiable goals with the employee's tangible personal goals and lays out a clear path for that person to achieve his or her goals. When employees feel that the workplace helps them reach their personal goals, they feel fulfilled and passionate, they stay in it for the long haul and they sing the organization's praises to all who will listen.

Inspire the team to get on board, and watch them sail the ship. If this sounds like a long shot, start by reading together *The 7 Habits of Highly Effective People*, by Stephen R. Covey, and promoting those principles to the team.

Today more than ever, providing the best possible work environment is paramount to enriching the organizational culture and attracting and retaining top-notch talent. Workplaces are pulling out all the stops: nap areas, meditation time, onsite massage/acupuncture/chiropractic care, take-what-you-like vacation policies, profit sharing, beyond-competitive health-care benefits, chef-prepared meals onsite, one-month sabbatical after five years tenure, exercise incentive programs, tuition assistance and more. These incentives sound expensive, but in the long run they pay off big time by keeping world-class employees.

Improve the culture with clear mission/vision/values that everyone can get behind, with quantifiable goals that tie to IDPs and with an amazing work environment. It's a spectacular thing when it all comes together – made easier with the *FLOURISH!* method.

HIRE RIGHT IN THE FIRST PLACE

You hear it all of the time: "It's hard to attract and keep great talent in the senior living industry." That's true for the competition as well, but hiring works better with an ironclad strategy.

Marketing starts from the inside out. The CEO has to articulate a clear vision and inspire the team. Management can spot, attract and keep amazing talent. The team wakes up wanting to come to work. Their enthusiasm ignites a spark for clients and families as they visit. Happy customers refer other happy customers. Satisfaction surveys validate what clients and families love about the organization. Marketing efforts reflect those attributes, the organization regularly delivers on them, and a virtuous cycle of loyalty begins to turn.

In her book, *Why Can't I Hire Good People? Lessons on How to Hire Better*, Beth Smith lays out 7 steps for finding great employees.

First, she writes, "Create an ideal candidate description." An ideal candidate embodies the organization's mission, vision and values with very little training or guidance. They just naturally "get it." The ideal candidate is a perfect fit with the organizational culture and is eager to perpetuate that goodness throughout the internal and external workings of the organization.

Only then, Smith says, can you develop the job description and the job advertisement, which are two distinct tools.

The job description details the responsibilities and duties.

The job ad markets the position to the target audience. In the senior living industry, too often job ads are written in an effort to quickly attract the right help. Very little regard is given to what will attract the right person to the job. Smith recommends, "Ask, what is the organization's mission, and who would be the best fit?" Describe both to a tee, and the right candidate will apply.

Finally, Smith advises, conduct three consecutive but separate interviews. The first will answer, "Can I work with this person?" The second will reveal, "Can they do the job?" And the third, "Are they passionate?" The candidate who aces all three is the best fit for the job.

When you have ace candidates filling the majority of the positions in the organization, they pack the power to market like no other external marketing effort can. Passion and loyalty among the internal team gives way to passion and loyalty among clients and referrers. There's no marketing budget big enough to surpass that value. When combined with the *FLOURISH!* method for marketing, this hiring strategy ensures promotional power from deep within the organization.

PUT EMPLOYEES FIRST

To remain successful, the healthiest aging services organizations invest in a sequential order of priority:

1. Cultivate an amazing team
2. Keep clients, families and referrers happy
3. Attract prospects

Any aging services organization that is facing a customer acquisition challenge most often does not have a marketing problem in isolation. They have issues in the preceding two areas first.

What do all three areas have in common? People.

Honor the people within the team by hiring right in the first place, providing a great work culture and offering training and coaching. Implement a strong rewards and incentives program for delivering excellent customer satisfaction. Train management to regularly thank those on the front lines. Be sure that each employee has an individual development plan (IDP), engaging him or her in striving for and reaching personal and professional goals.

When employees feel honored by the organization, they are empowered to honor the clients and families. Fulfilled employees genuinely listen to the needs of clients and families, ensuring they feel like they belong and giving them what they want, over and over and over again.

Beyond that, fulfilled employees honor prospects by showing up in places they frequent, listening to their needs, being of service (through kindness or education) without expecting immediate compensation and guiding them toward making the best possible next choice in finding a solution.

Fulfilled employees do all of this naturally, with little prompting from management.

And they are delighted to learn and deploy strategies like the *FLOURISH!* method because they believe in their organization.

RATCHET UP THE REFERRAL "ASK"

Inevitably, referrals trickle in from time to time by virtue of the aging services organization's reputation. The trick to growing word-of-mouth is to systematize the process of attracting referrals to a momentum of steady inquiries.

Three things matter: List, Ask, Remind.

List
Work with the team to make a list of those people who are most likely to refer. Include the names of current clients, their families and healthcare providers that have sent referrals in the past. Then cast a wider net, jotting down the names of people and entities that may refer if prompted.

For smaller organizations, make it a point for someone to connect once a week in a meaningful way with each name on the list. Small gestures go a long way. For example, comment about a post on a referring family member's personal Facebook page. Send a referring healthcare provider a book, article or other educational item of interest. Take a referring practitioner out for coffee or lunch. Send a referring organization a basket of fruit to thank them. Take individuals who refer most often to a local sporting event. These tactics keep you top-of-mind, which is the heart of marketing.

The premise is the same for larger organizations; however, the scale is bigger. Content marketing takes the place of one-on-one conversations, serving up educational articles straight to referrers' inboxes. The more valuable the knowledge, the more likely the recipient is to forward or share the message. Social media marketing and events cast a wider call for referrals. The 80/20 rule goes for events, too. Share 80% of the time about general social things that loosely reflect the organization's values, and 20% of the time be promotional by asking for referrals.

Another idea is to reward referrers with a gift card or other diversion that reflects the organization's Message and Design Equation.

Regardless of the size of the organization, create systems and structures to ensure that a mailed, handwritten thank-you note goes to anyone who refers. Ask the referrer how you can help them then deliver on their request. The most valuable appreciation you can give is to connect a referrer with other people who can in turn help them.

Ask

Train yourself and the team to be alert to moments when clients or their families compliment the organization or staff. This is a door opening. It's the heart softening. It's that rare moment of true connection between two human beings.

It is the best moment for the team member to casually yet clearly deliver a referral question.

The golden rule in marketing is simple yet complex: *People must be told exactly what to do in order for them to act.* This is especially true in asking for referrals.

There are many ways to ask and team members need to be ready with a phrase that feels right. Here are a few examples:

"We love your dad. We'd love to care for your other older friends and family who will benefit from our services. Please send them our way."

Or, "It's our pleasure. Please keep us in mind for others you may know."

Or simply, "Thank you. Please refer us."

Reward
The "ask" is an acquired skill. It takes time and lots of practice. Role-play in team meetings so it becomes a comfortable communication for everyone. Hold regular team trainings to keep staff ready to ask on a regular basis. Reward those who ask most frequently, which is measured by the highest number of referrals in a quarter.

Reward clients and families who refer with a simple thank you note, a gift card to a nice restaurant or other appropriate gesture of gratitude.

***

Get ready with a professional presentation to the medical industry. Healthcare practitioners, hospitals and home care agencies are always looking for reputable aging services organizations to which to refer their patients. A simple PowerPoint will suffice to showcase professional credentials and success stories. Consider sending a link to an online referral form to professional referrers, reminding them to refer and making it easy for them to do so.

When new inquiries start to drop off, that's the time to reexamine the referral system. Recalibrating this system is the easiest, least expensive way to jumpstart new business. Resist the temptation to spend time and money attracting new inquiries from other sources first. And skip investing in expensive professional referral services that send less-than-ideal leads they haven't qualified through your survey of desired clients. The referred resident or family member who is cultivated from your team and culture is more readily attracted to the organization, is more likely to sign on as a resident and is most likely to love what you have to offer.

Talk about tapping the *FLOURISH!* method.

POWERFULLY ALIGN SALES AND MARKETING

The resident and family are buying a *relationship* with your aging services organization. Not a bed. Not care. Not safety. Not even peace of mind. A relationship.

That said, every great relationship is built on a strong foundation of listening. There are only two requirements for listening:

1. Ask open-ended, thought-provoking and targeted questions to get to the heart of the matter. (In great marketing, the first step is to ask the right questions. So it is with sales.)
2. Talk only 10% of the time. Make eye contact and hear what the individual is saying the rest of the time. Less is more. Resist the inclination to describe the features and benefits. The key is to get at the heart of their individual situation *first*, then work *together* to create a solution to meet those desires.

Here are a few questions, adapted from the book, *Being Mortal*, by Atul Gawande to help both the team member and the inquiring party get a full picture of the reality of the situation:

- What is your understanding of your mother's situation?
- What is your understanding of the potential outcome if we proceed?
- What is your understanding of the potential outcome if we *do not* proceed?
- What are your mother's hopes? Fears?
- What are your hopes? Fears?

It is always appropriate to ask, "Why is that important to you?" This allows the prospect to be vulnerable. It also helps them to articulate what motivates them. Both are key in building the relationship and converting the prospect into an actual client.

The next series of questions help ascertain how ready they are to proceed:

- What compromise is your mother willing to make? Not willing to make?
- What compromise are you willing to make? Not willing to make?
- When things go extremely well, what will she/you accomplish?
- What is the impact of this on her/your quality of life right now?
- Based upon all of that knowledge, what is the course of action that best serves your family?

These questions conclude with the action question: "Are you ready for the next step?" Train the staff that the goal is not to get the prospect to sign yet, but to *take the next step*. That could be to take a tour, meet the team or agree to an assessment. The staff member will ask this question multiple times throughout the sales process, moving the prospect closer and closer to the ultimate action of becoming a client, one step at a time.

The next set of questions helps clarify the financials:

- What is your understanding of how much this will cost?
- Would you be interested in seeing a cost/benefit analysis?
- How would you prefer to pay?
- If money were not a factor, how would you proceed?

Finally, two questions help solidify the relationship, make a commitment and complete the conversation:

- Would you like to see a written lease agreement with payment details?
- Are you ready to sign?

When the answers come from the hearts of the clients and families, the *FLOURISH!* method naturally and powerfully aligns sales and marketing efforts.

TOP 10 MISTAKES IN INTERNAL MARKETING

1. **Neglect.** When inquiries drop off, few aging services organizations think to ratchet up internal marketing at first.

2. **Not being the change.** If the organization is in need of a culture shift, but you are not in a position of leadership, or otherwise don't believe that you can be the catalyst to change, think again. Initiate the change that you wish to see in your organization. A great place to start is by taking notes from *The 7 Habits of Highly Effective People*, by Stephen R. Covey, and sharing them with your team.

3. **Dart-in-the-dark hiring.** Minimize turnover and maximize morale by hiring right in the first place. Hit the bullseye with a strategy like the one in *Why Can't I Hire Good People? Lessons on How to Hire Better*, by Beth Smith.

4. **Training but not inspiring.** The team is the most valable asset. Go beyond teaching them. Excite them!

5. **Going it alone.** Every aspect of internal marketing should be deployed by a team. Go beyond becoming a great leader yourself. Empower teammates to become leaders, too.

6. **Failing to ask.** You have to solicit referrals. If you want people to take action, tell them specifically what you want them to do.

7. **Leaning on referral services.** Stop investing in expensive referral services that send less-than-ideal leads. A lead cultivated from referral is much more valuable.

8. **Talking too much.** Listen rather than present in the sales process. Listening builds relationships.

9. **Going for the close too early.** At the appropriate moment, invite prospects to take the next logical step toward becoming clients, and they will naturally come to a point of committing. Don't rush it, lest they think you're too pushy.

10. **Waiting too long.** Rather than waiting for referrals to trickle in spontaneously, systematize the process of attracting them for stability and steady growth.

AFTERWORD

We have entered an Age of Fear in healthcare.

Fear of encroaching competitors. Fear of the shift to digital marketing. Fear that the Affordable Care Act (or the evolution away from it) will cost us dearly. Fear of the trending consolidation of providers.

The word "science," is Latin for "knowledge." Ralph Waldo Emerson said, "Knowledge is the antidote for fear."

The more knowledge you gain about marketing, the easier you will find a cure for these fears. You will benefit from a cure that allows you to attract warm leads, people who are ready to commit to your organization and help it thrive. You can stand out in even the most saturated of markets.

More than that, you can concentrate on changing the things that will make your profession easier and more rewarding. Thanks to the *FLOURISH!* method of simplifying the process of getting the best marketing results, you can finally focus on what matters most: the life-changing services you offer to older adults.

EXERCISE 1

YOUR MESSAGE AND DESIGN EQUATION

Use this exercise to formulate the Message and Design Equation.

1. What are three ways clients and families say this organization is different and better than competitors? (Be sure these are benefits, not features. Gentle care is a benefit. Memory care is a feature. Each item should be objective and, where possible, quantifiable. Think, "Residents are warmly greeted by three team members before 9 a.m. every day," as opposed to, "Residents think the team is nice.")

o _____

o _____

o _____

2. What is the No. 1 attribute people like best about the organization? (It's usually the benefit that comes up over and over again in survey responses. If you keep seeing "funny," "laughter" and "smiling" in the survey responses, the No. 1 attribute may be "humor." Remember, clients and families are often drawn in by *non-clinical* benefits. They are buying a relationship with you, not just expertise.)

Message: _____

Design:
(Describe below, in writing or as a collage of pictures, the types of imagery, illustration, photography, etc., that best represent your message.)

EXERCISE 2

YOUR BALANCED MARKETING FORMULA

Use this exercise to formulate your Balanced Marketing Formula. Download a larger copy at www.bloommarketinginc.com/flourish.

AVAILABLE MARKETING BUDGET: _____
AVERAGE NEW RESIDENT VALUE: _____
TOTAL EXPECTED ROI: _____
TOTAL ACTUAL ROI: _____

TACTIC: _____
PARTY RESPONSIBLE: _____
MARKETING BUDGET: _____
EXPECTED ROI: _____
ACTUAL ROI: _____

TACTIC: _____
PARTY RESPONSIBLE: _____
MARKETING BUDGET: _____
EXPECTED ROI: _____
ACTUAL ROI: _____

BRAND AWARENESS

TRADITIONAL MARKETING

ONLINE MARKETING

INTERNAL MARKETING

TACTIC: _____
PARTY RESPONSIBLE: _____
MARKETING BUDGET: _____
EXPECTED ROI: _____
ACTUAL ROI: _____

TACTIC: _____
PARTY RESPONSIBLE: _____
MARKETING BUDGET: _____
EXPECTED ROI: _____
ACTUAL ROI: _____

SAMPLE BALANCED MARKETING FORMULA

Use this sample to guide you in formulating your organization's Balanced Marketing Formula.

Download a larger copy at www.bloommarketinginc.com/flourish.

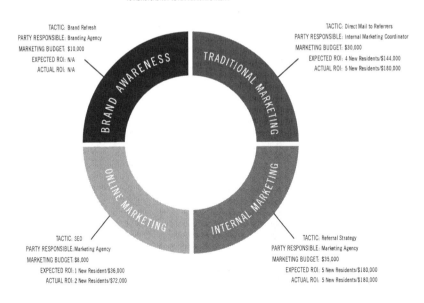

AVAILABLE MARKETING BUDGET: $83,000
AVERAGE NEW RESIDENT VALUE: $3,000/mo. or $36,000/yr.
TOTAL EXPECTED ROI: 10 New Residents/$360,000
TOTAL ACTUAL ROI: 12 New Residents/$432,000

TACTIC: Brand Refresh
PARTY RESPONSIBLE: Branding Agency
MARKETING BUDGET: $10,000
EXPECTED ROI: N/A
ACTUAL ROI: N/A

TACTIC: Direct Mail to Referrers
PARTY RESPONSIBLE: Internal Marketing Coordinator
MARKETING BUDGET: $30,000
EXPECTED ROI: 4 New Residents/$144,000
ACTUAL ROI: 5 New Residents/$180,000

TACTIC: SEO
PARTY RESPONSIBLE: Marketing Agency
MARKETING BUDGET: $8,000
EXPECTED ROI: 1 New Resident/$36,000
ACTUAL ROI: 2 New Residents/$72,000

TACTIC: Referral Strategy
PARTY RESPONSIBLE: Marketing Agency
MARKETING BUDGET: $35,000
EXPECTED ROI: 5 New Residents/$180,000
ACTUAL ROI: 5 New Residents/$180,000

BRAND AWARENESS

TRADITIONAL MARKETING

ONLINE MARKETING

INTERNAL MARKETING

STAY ON THE CUTTING EDGE

Liked what you read and want more?

Get more thought-provoking insights directly from Wendy O'Donovan Phillips with no additional cost. Here are two easy ways you can receive timely and relevant content updates that build upon the *FLOURISH!* method and guide the organization:

1. Go to www.bloommarketinginc.com/blog and enter your email address to receive regular content updates.
2. Like us on Facebook at www.facebook.com/bloommarketinginc to get regular content updates in your social newsfeed.

All content is crafted exclusively by Wendy and her team to promote change and growth in your organization.

ACKNOWLEDGMENTS

Many people helped make this book. My dad, Bill O'Donovan, is the reason I am in communications; having spent four decades in the newspaper industry, he has instilled in me a love for the written word and a passion for the art of persuasion. He edited this book. To quote Mary Baker Eddy, he was at once "wise and gentle and strong and fearless" in his editing, as he is in his fathering.

My mom, Bonnie O'Donovan, has been my staunch supporter throughout my life and career. Too, she demonstrated excellence in healthcare to me, having worked for four decades in the industry.

My husband, Trevor Lee Phillips, has always stood by me and cheered me on, even when my marketing agency and this book were mere pipe dreams. I get to check "write a book" off my bucket list thanks to his advocacy. I am grateful to him also for caring for our daughter, Willa, late at night and on weekends while I wrote.

My team members at work are the best leaders I know: Melinda Gisbert, Molly Watkins, Alex Garcia, Chelsea Humbach, Casey Schmidt and Stephanie Vecchiarelli. Melinda inspired the contents of the book and helped to edit and proof it. Molly project managed the book. Stephanie expertly laid out the design. They all impeccably held down the agency while I was writing.

Alicia Marie provided the coaching that has led me here and the inspiration for the section on culture. Brenda Abdilla kept me calm, and Mary LoVerde provided mentorship and manuscript feedback. Many professionals let me learn from their example: Alan Wyngarden, Debbie Lovill, Lisa Stemmer, Ryan Wilson and more.

I'm lucky to have each one of you in my corner.

73538017R00075

Made in the USA
San Bernardino, CA
07 April 2018